TABLE OF CONTENTS

OVERVIEW……………………………….......3

HOW TO LOSE WEIGHT FAST……………….....5

TEN WEIGHTLOSS TIPS………………………...15

HOW TO LOSE WEIGHT ON A DEADLINE……….20

TIPS TO MEASURE AND CONTROL PORTION SIZES………………………………………………28

HOW TO CONTROL YOUR PORTION SIZE....…….43

BENEFITS OF PORTION CONTROL BEYOND WEIGHT LOSS……………………………..…..47

THE LIFESTYLE CHANGE……………………....58

OVERVIEW

This diet plan is based on portion control, coupled with minimal effort exercise, and smarter choices of the foods you eat now. This is the easiest diet to stay on and is designed to help you lose weight, and I guarantee it.

If you follow the plan, you will succeed, as the equation for losing weight is mathematical. For instance, if the average daily intake of calories is 4000, and you adjust your intake (calorie count) to 3000, you will lose weight proportionately. If you adjust your intake and exercise, you can fine-tune your weight loss to an optimum rate, while any improvements in the food choices you make affect the overall success.

Anyone can use this system, but I designed it for folks who are "heavy," like myself, and would like to lose over fifty pounds. If you are looking to lose less than fifty pounds, you should not start this system; instead, review the first 32 pages of this book and develop your own best method based on individual foods' caloric value.

This weight loss system is designed for long-term use and is entirely adjustable to meet your needs. You should refer to the first 32 pages of this book for a guide for references and data to help you on your way to looking and feeling great. To begin the diet, you will not be so fast to quit; go to page 34.

HOW TO LOSE WEIGHT FAST

There are many ways to lose a lot of weight fast. That said, many diet plans leave you feeling hungry or unsatisfied. These are major reasons why you might find it hard to stick to a diet. However, not all diets have this effect. Unfortunately, this, is the diet most people fail at. Low carb diets are effective for weight loss and may be easier to stick to than other diets, but without the motivation, you won't stick with it, so, it won't work.

Here's a traditional 3-step weight loss plan that employs a low carb diet and aims to:

Significantly reduce your appetite cause fast weight loss to improve your metabolic health at the same time

Cut back on carbs

The most important part is to cut back on sugars and starches or carbohydrates.

When you do that, your hunger levels go down, and you generally end up eating significantly fewer calories Instead of burning carbs for energy, your body now starts burning stored fat for energy.

Another benefit of cutting carbs is that it lowers insulin levels, causing the kidneys to shed excess sodium and water. This reduces bloating and unnecessary water weight. According to some dietitians, it's not uncommon to lose up to 10 pounds (4.5 kg) — sometimes more — in the first week of eating this way. This weight loss includes both body fat and water weight.

One study in healthy women with obesity reported that a very low carb diet was more effective than a low-fat diet for short-term weight loss.

Research suggests that a low carb diet can reduce appetite, leading you to eat fewer calories without thinking about it or feeling hungry. Put simply, reducing carbs can lead to quick, easy weight loss.

Summary

Removing sugars and starches or carbs from your diet can reduce your appetite, lower your insulin levels, and cause you to lose weight without feeling hungry. However, without the motivation to continue, chances are very low, it will work for you.

Eat protein, fat, and vegetables

Each one of your meals should include a protein source, fat Source, and low carb vegetables.

As, a general rule, try eating two to three meals per day. If you find yourself hungry in the afternoon, add a fourth meal.

Constructing your meals in this way should bring your carb intake down to around 20–50 grams per day.

To see how you can assemble your meals, check out this low carb meal plan and list 101 healthy low carb recipes.

Protein

Eating plenty of protein is an essential part of this plan. Evidence suggests that eating lots of protein may boost calorie expenditure by 80–100 calories per day.

High protein diets can also reduce cravings and obsessive thoughts about food by 60%, reduce the desire to snack late at night by half, and make you feel full. In one study, people on a higher protein diet ate 441 fewer calories per days.

When it comes to losing weight, protein is a crucial nutrient to think about. Healthy protein sources include:
- Meat: beef, chicken, pork, and lamb
- Fish and seafood: salmon, trout, and shrimp

- Eggs: Whole eggs with the yolk
- Plant-based proteins: beans, legumes, and soy

Low carb vegetables

Don't be afraid to load your plate with low carb vegetables. They are packed with nutrients, and you can eat very large amounts without going over 20–50 net carbs per day. A diet based mostly on lean protein sources and vegetables contains all the fiber, vitamins, and minerals you need to be healthy.

Many vegetables are low in carbs, including:

- broccoli
- cauliflower
- spinach
- tomatoes
- kale
- Brussels sprouts
- cabbage

- Swiss chard
- lettuce
- cucumber

Healthy fats

Don't be afraid of eating fats. Trying to do low carb and low fat at the same time can make sticking to the diet very difficult. Sources of healthy fats include:

- olive oil
- coconut oil
- avocado oil
- butter

Summary

Assemble each meal out of a protein source, fat Source, and low carb vegetables. This will generally put you in a carb range of 20–50 grams and significantly lower your hunger levels.

Lift weights three times per week

You don't need to exercise to lose weight on this plan, but it will have extra benefits.

By lifting weights, you will burn lots of calories and prevent your metabolism from slowing down, which is a common side effect of losing weight.

Studies on low carb diets show that you can gain muscle while losing significant amounts of body fat.

Try going to the gym three to four times a week to lift weights. If you're new to the gym, ask a trainer for some advice.

If lifting weights is not an option for you, doing some cardio workouts like walking, jogging, running, cycling, or swimming will suffice. Both cardio and weightlifting can help with weight loss.

Summary

Resistance training, such as weight lifting, maybe the best option. If that's not possible, cardio workouts are also effective.

Try Doing A 'Carb Refeed' Once Per Week

If you need to, you can take one day off per week where you eat more carbs. Many people choose to do this on Saturday. It's important to stick to healthy carb sources like oats, rice, quinoa, potatoes, sweet potatoes, and fruit. If you must have a cheat meal and eat something unhealthy, do it on this day. Limit this to one higher carb day per week. If you aren't reducing carbs enough, you might not experience weight loss.

You might gain some water weight during your refeed day, and you will generally lose it again in the next 1–2 days.

Summary

Having one day each week where you eat more carbs is acceptable, although not necessary.

What about calories and portion control?

It's unnecessary to count calories as long as you keep your carb intake very low and stick to protein, fat, and low carb vegetables.

However, if you want to count them, you can use a free online calculator like this one.

Enter your sex, weight, height, and activity levels. The calculator will tell you how many calories to eat per day to maintain your weight, lose weight, or lose weight fast.

You can also download free, easy-to-use calorie counters from websites and app stores. Here is a list of 5 calorie counters to try.

Summary

It's not necessary to count calories to lose weight on this plan. It's most important to keep your carbs in the 20–50-gram range strictly.

TEN WEIGHT LOSS TIPS

Eat a high protein breakfast. Eating a high protein breakfast could reduce cravings and calorie intake throughout the day.

Avoid sugary drinks and fruit juice. These are among the most fattening things you can put into your body.

Drink water before meals. One study showed that drinking water a half hour before meals increased weight loss by 44% over three months .

Choose weight-loss-friendly foods. Some foods are better for weight loss than others. Here is a list of 20 healthy weight-loss-friendly foods.

Eat soluble fiber. Studies show that soluble fibers may promote weight loss. Fiber supplements like glucomannan can also help.

Drink coffee or tea. Caffeine boosts your metabolism by 3–11%.

Base your diet on whole foods. They are healthier, more filling, and much less likely to cause overeating than processed foods.

Eat slowly. Eating quickly can lead to weight gain over time, while eating slowly makes you feel more full and boosts weight-reducing hormones.

Weigh yourself every day. Studies show that people who weigh themselves every day are much more likely to lose weight and keep it off for a long time.

Get good quality sleep. Sleep is important for many reasons, and poor sleep is one of the biggest risk factors for weight gain (30).

For more tips on weight loss, read about 30 natural tips for losing weight here.

Summary

Sticking to the three-step plan allows for quick weight loss, and using other tips will make the diet plan even more effective.

How Fast Will You Lose Weight?

You may lose 5–10 pounds (2.3–4.5 kg) of weight — sometimes more — in the first week of the diet plan and then lose weight consistently after that.

If you're new to dieting, weight loss may happen more quickly. The more weight you have to lose, the faster you will lose it.

For the first few days, you might feel a bit strange. Your body is used to running off carbs, and it can take time for it to get used to burning fat instead.

Some people experience the "keto flu" or "low carb flu." It's usually over within a few days.

After the first few days, most people report feeling very good, with even more energy than before.

Aside from weight loss, the low carb diet can improve your health in many ways:

- blood sugar levels tend to decrease on low carb diets (31) significantly
- triglycerides tend to go down
- LDL (bad) cholesterol goes down
- HDL (good) cholesterol goes up
- blood pressure improves significantly
- low carb diets can be as easy to follow as low-fat diets

Summary

Most people lose a significant amount of weight on a low carb diet, but the speed depends on the individual. Low carb diets also improve certain markers of health, such as blood sugar and cholesterol levels.

The bottom line

By reducing carbs and lowering insulin levels, you'll likely experience reduced appetite and hunger. This removes the main reasons it's often difficult to maintain a weight loss plan.

You can likely eat healthy food on this plan until you're full and still lose a significant amount of fat. The initial drop in water weight can lead to a drop in the scales within a few days. Fat loss takes longer.

Studies comparing low carb and low-fat diets suggest that a low carb diet might even make you lose up to two to three times as much weight as a typical low fat, calorie-restricted diet.

If you have type 2 diabetes, talk to your healthcare provider before making changes, as this plan can reduce your need for medication

HOW TO LOSE WEIGHT ON A DEADLINE

If you want to lose 10 pounds fast, you don't have time to start a diet delivery plan, hire a personal trainer, or read self-help books. You need a no-nonsense approach that accomplishes two basic things:

Burns more calories than you consume

Provides ample nutrition irrespective of the calorie count

The bottom line is that you want to be both sensible and realistic in your approach. While some people can shed 10 pounds in a few weeks, the amount you lose ultimately depends on your starting weight, your current health and age, and your commitment to a holistic plan involving diet and exercise.

Establish Your Goals and Intentions

To begin, start by outlining why you want to lose weight. If it is because you're preparing for an event or are simply tired of carrying around the extra pounds, write it down on paper. As basic as this may seem, it sets your intention and allows you to evaluate your goals objectively.

If you aim to fit into a size six dress in time for your high school reunion, you can assess how realistic that goal is within the prescribed time frame. On the other hand, if you are simply fed up and want to lose weight now, you may want to take another look at your intentions. It is also important to discuss your plans with your healthcare provider to confirm whether your goals are healthy.

Often, if you steamroll into a weight-loss plan, you will quickly lose steam if you don't reach your magic number fast (this is also why a "magic number" may not be a helpful goal). By establishing your goals from the start, you can assess how attainable they are and what you need to achieve them. Also, know that diets are not sustainable for long-term change.

Healthy weight loss occurs at a rate of around one to two pounds per week.1 Most experts will tell you that losing anything more is unwise, increasing the risk of nutritional deficiencies, muscle loss, hair loss, and menstrual irregularities.

Calculate How Many Calories You Usually Eat

Weight loss is all about consuming fewer calories than you burn during routine activity. The best way to figure this out is by writing down everything you eat in a day.

Since you're on a deadline, you won't have time to keep a food diary to track your intake over a week. Instead, just sit down and crunch the numbers, listing everything you eat and drink on a normal day. You can then use a nutritional counter to add how many calories you consume in 24 hours.

Try not to pad the list with indulgent foods you only eat occasionally. The goal is to get your baseline intake so that you can determine exactly how many calories you need to cut back.

Calculate How Many Calories You Need to Cut

An average woman needs to consume about 2,000 calories per day to maintain a normal weight and 1,500 calories to lose one pound per week. An average man needs around 2,500 and 2,000 calories, respectively, to do the same.

If you are overweight, you are likely to consume more than this. As such, it would be unrealistic to think you can suddenly drop from 3,500 calories to 1,500 calories per day and remain healthy. You won't. This is especially true if you are older, are largely inactive, or have medical conditions to manage.

To this end, use an online weight loss calculator to determine how many calories you need to cut back on based on your age, height, current weight, activity level, and target date. The calculator will tell you if your weight loss goals are too ambitious and likely put you at risk.

Never consume fewer than 1,200 calories per day if you're a woman or 1,500 calories per day if you're a man. For some people, even these figures are too aggressive.

Create Your Diet Plan

Now that you've done your initial calculations, you can subtract the recommended caloric intake from the number of calories you currently consume. For example, if you currently consume 2,800 calories per day and need to eat no more than 2,000 to lose a pound or two per week, that leaves you with 800 calories to cut.

But rather than just saying, "I'll cut out all bread," take the time to build a weekly menu that is balanced and meets your daily nutritional needs. While you can certainly take a daily supplement, it is far better to get your food nutrients.

According to the 2015-2020 Dietary Guidelines for Americans issued by the U.S. Department of Agriculture, a balanced diet should contain ample quantities of vegetables, fruits, beans, grains (whole and refined) and moderate amounts of chicken, fish, lean meat, and low-fat dairy.2

On top of that, no more than 15 to 29 grams of oil (unsaturated and polyunsaturated) should be consumed per day. Less than 10% of calories should come from added sugars and less than 10% from saturated fats.

Get Active

If you want to meet your weight loss goal within a specific time frame, you cannot do it without exercise. Remember that the weight-loss equation is based on burning more calories than you consume. By increasing your activity level, even by as little as 10 minutes per day, you will be burning calories faster than you did when you first started.

Start with a simple five-minute routine and make an effort to increase the intensity and duration of your workout every week. This is a realistic approach that helps develop a lifelong habit you can maintain once your weight loss goal is met. By keeping active, you will begin to see results before you know it a little every day.

But don't overdo it. Over-exercising is likely to put you on the fast track to injury, not weight loss. Take a day or two off per week to give your muscles a chance to recover, strengthen, and grow after strenuous activity. On your days off, enjoy a walk with a friend and do other activities you enjoy to reward yourself.

Track Your Progress

While most of us measure our weight loss by stepping on the scale, it is equally important to keep track of the tools for weight loss, namely the number of calories you eat and the amount of activity you put in.

TIPS TO MEASURE AND CONTROL PORTION SIZES

Obesity is a growing epidemic, as more people than ever are struggling to control their weight.

Increased portion sizes are thought to contribute to overeating and unwanted weight gain.

People tend to eat almost all of what they serve themselves. Therefore, controlling portion sizes can help prevent overindulging. Here are nine tips for measuring and control portion sizes — both at home and on the go.

Use Smaller Dinnerware

Evidence suggests that sizes of plates, spoons and glasses can unconsciously influence how much food someone eats.

For example, using large plates can make food appear smaller — often leading to overeating.

In one study, people using a large bowl ate 77% more pasta than those using a medium-sized bowl.

In another study, nutritional experts served themselves 31% more ice cream than larger bowls and 14.5% more when provided with larger serving spoons.

Interestingly, most people who ate more due to large dishes were completely unaware of the portion size.

Therefore, swapping your usual plate, bowl or serving spoon for a smaller alternative can reduce the helping of food and prevent overeating.

Most people feel just as full having eaten from a smaller dish as from a large one

Summary

Simply using smaller dishes or glasses can lower the amount of food or drink you consume. What's more, people teSnd to feel just as satisfied.

Use Your Plate as a Portion Guide

If measuring or weighing food isn't appealing, try using your plate or bowl as a portion control guide.

This can help you determine the optimal macronutrient ratio for a well-balanced meal.

A rough guide for each meal is:

Vegetables or salad: Half a plate

High-quality protein: Quarter of a plate — this includes meat, poultry, fish, eggs, dairy, tofu, beans and pulses

Complex carbs: Quarter of a plate — such as whole grains and starchy vegetables

High-fat foods: Half a tablespoon (7 grams) — including cheese, oils and butter

Remember that this is a rough guide, as people have different dietary needs. For example, those who are more physically active often require more food.

As vegetables and salad are naturally low in calories but high in fiber and other nutrients, filling up on these may help you avoid overeating calorie-dense foods.

If you want extra guidance, some manufacturers sell portion-control plates.

Summary

Using a plate as a guide for portion control can help you curb total food intake. You can divide your plate into sections based on different food groups.

Use Your Hands as a Serving Guide

Another way to gauge the appropriate portion size without any measuring tools is by simply using your hands.

As your hands usually correspond to your body size, bigger people who require more food typically have bigger hands (8Trusted Source).

A rough guide for each meal is:

High-protein foods: A palm-sized serving for women and two palm-sized portions for men — such as meat, fish, poultry and beans

Vegetables and salads: A fist-sized portion for women and two fist-sized portions for men

High-carb foods: One cupped-hand portion for women and two for men — such as whole grains and starchy vegetables

High-fat foods: One thumb-sized portion for women and two for men — such as butter, oils and nuts

Summary

Your hands can be a helpful guide for portion sizes. Different food groups correspond to various shapes and parts of your hands.

Ask for a Half Portion When Eating Out

Restaurant serving sizes are, on average, about 2.5 times larger than standard serving sizes — and up to a whopping eight times larger. If you are eating out, you can always ask for a half or a children's dish.

This will save you a lot of calories and help prevent overeating

Alternatively, you could share a meal with someone or order a starter and side instead of the main dish. Other tips include ordering a side salad or vegetables, asking for sauces and dressings to be served separately and avoiding buffet-style. In this all-you-can-eat restaurants, it's very easy to overindulge.

Summary

Restaurant portions tend to be at least twice the size of a regular portion. Prevent overeating by asking for a half portion, ordering a starter instead of the main dish and avoiding buffet-style restaurants.

Start All Meals With a Glass of Water

Drinking a glass of water up to 30 minutes before a meal will naturally aid portion control.

Filling up on water will make you feel less hungry. Being well hydrated also helps you distinguish between hunger and thirst.

One study in middle-aged and older adults observed that drinking 17 ounces (500 ml) of water before each meal resulted in a 44% greater decline in weight over 12 weeks, most likely due to reduced food intake.

Similarly, when overweight and obese older adults drank 17 ounces (500 ml) of water 30 minutes before a meal, they consumed 13% fewer calories without trying to make any changes.

In another study in young normal-weight men, drinking a similar amount of water immediately before a meal resulted in greater feelings of fullness and reduced food intake.

Therefore, having a glass of water before each meal can help prevent overeating and aid portion control.

Summary

Drinking a glass of water up to 30 minutes before a meal can naturally result in reduced food intake and greater fullness feelings.

Take It Slowly

Eating quickly makes you less aware of getting full — and therefore increases your likelihood of overeating.

As your brain can take around 20 minutes to register that you are full after eating, slowing down can reduce your total intake.

For example, one study in healthy women noted that eating slowly led to greater feelings of fullness and decreased food intake than eating quickly.

What's more, the women who ate slowly tended to enjoy their meal more.

Also, eating on the go or while distracted or watching TV boosts your likelihood of overeating.

Therefore, focusing on your meal and refusing to rush increases the chances you'll enjoy it and control your portion sizes.

Health experts recommend taking smaller bites and chewing every mouthful at least five or six times before swallowing.

Summary

Sitting down to meals with no other distractions and eating slowly will regulate portion control and reduce your overeating likelihood.

Don't Eat Straight From the Container

Jumbo-size packages or food served from large containers encourages overeating and less awareness of appropriate portion sizes.

This is especially true for snacks.

Evidence suggests that people tend to eat more out of large packages than small ones — regardless of food taste or quality.

For example, people ate 129% more candies when served from a large container than a small one.

In another study, participants consumed over 180 fewer grams of snacks per week when given 100-gram snack packs than when given snacks in standard-sized packages.

Rather than eating snacks from the original packaging, empty them into a small bowl to prevent eating more than you need.

The same applies to bulk portions of family meals. Rather than serving food directly from the stove, re-portion it onto plates before serving. Doing so will help prevent overfilling your plate and discourage returning for seconds.

Summary

Eating food from larger packages or containers encourages increased intake. Try re-portioning snacks into individual portions and serving family meals from plates to prevent overeating.

Be Aware of Suitable Serving Size

Research indicates that we can't always rely on our judgment of the appropriate portion size.

This is because many factors affect portion control.

However, it may help to invest in a scale or measuring cup to weigh food and correctly assess your intake.

Reading food labels also increases awareness of proper portions.

Knowing recommended serving sizes for commonly eaten foods can help you moderate your intake.

Here are some examples:

- Cooked pasta or rice: 1/2 cup (75 and 100 grams, respectively)
- Vegetables and salad: 1–2 cups (150–300 grams)
- Breakfast cereal: 1 cup (40 grams)
- Cooked beans: 1/2 cup (90 grams)
- Nut butter: 2 tablespoons (16 grams)
- Cooked meats: 3 ounces (85 grams)

You don't always have to measure your meals. However, doing so may help a short period develop an awareness of what an appropriate portion size looks like. After a while, you may not need to measure everything.

Summary

Using measuring equipment can help increase portion sizes and correctly assess how much food is normally eaten.

Use a Food Diary

Research suggests that people are often surprised at how much food they eat.

For example, one study found that 21% of people who ate more due to having larger serving bowls denied having eaten more (21).

Writing down all food and drink intake can increase awareness of the type and amount of foods you're consuming.

Those who kept a food diary in weight-loss studies tended to lose more weight overall (22).

This likely occurred because they became more aware of what they ate — including their unhealthy choices — and adjusted their diet accordingly.

Summary

Jotting down your total calorie intake can increase awareness of what you consume. This can motivate you to make healthier choices and reduce your chances of overeating.

The Bottom Line

However, there are many practical steps you can take to control portions. These simple changes have proven successful in reducing portions without compromising on taste or feelings of fullness.

For example, measuring your food, using smaller dishes, drinking water before meals and eating slowly can all reduce your risk of overeating. Portion control is a quick fix that improves your quality of life and may prevent binging.

HOW TO CONTROL YOUR PORTION SIZE

Switching to smaller plates, meal prepping and using kitchen gadgets are some of the simple solutions to help healthy eaters control their portion size.

Measure Accurately

It might seem time-consuming to correctly measure out the exact milliliters of oil or a portion of pasta by tablespoon, but it's still the most accurate way to work out your serving size.

Use Your Hands

Measuring portion size against your hands is a quick and precise alternative to using weighing scales. For example, a portion of meat or poultry is roughly the size of your palm;

cheese works out the size of about two thumbs, and a portion of fruit should fit the size of your fist.

Use Small Plates

Overeating can often be attributed to the size of the plate you are serving on, as the larger the surface, the more likely you are to try and fill it. Smaller plates will make your meals appear larger, helping you to reduce excessively big portions.

Gadget Up

If you are prepared to spend a little cash to help work out your food helpings, then there are plenty of useful gadgets that can help. Tools such as portion scoops, spaghetti measurers and portion plates are most ideal.

Stick To The 20-Minute Rule

If you still feel hungry after eating, make sure to leave at least 20 minutes for your food to settle before going back for seconds. This will give you time to digest the food you've already eaten and should help put a stop to any feelings of hunger.

Gauge When You're Full

Making sure you don't overeat means making sure you don't eat until you're full. Try to gauge when you feel about 70-80% full and then stop. Otherwise, you'll end up gorging on far more than your recommended number of portions.

Meal-Prep For Accurate Portion Size

Preparing your lunch and dinners in advance allows you to measure out an appropriate portion size for each meal, saving you from the temptation to cook excessive amounts of food when it comes to eating.

Avoid Cooking Leftovers

Cooking extra food that can be saved for another meal might seem like a good time-saving idea, but you run the risk of giving in to your hunger and eating it all in one sitting. Only make what you want to eat there and then; otherwise, you'll end up overheating.

Don't Skip Meals

Skipping meals will only serve to make you feel hungrier once you do decide to eat, and the more ravenous you feel when cooking, the more likely it is that you'll bite off more food than you can chew.

BENEFITS OF PORTION CONTROL BEYOND WEIGHT LOSS

When it comes to losing weight — or just healthy eating in general — the rules around food are pretty simple: Don't overeat, control your portion sizes and listen to your body's fullness cues.

But knowing the guidelines and putting them into practice are two different things, and the latter can be a lot more difficult — especially when that extra-large slice of chocolate cake is staring you down.

Controlling your portion sizes isn't just lip service, though; there are some real benefits, both physically and financially, when it comes to dialing down the amount you're piling on your plate.

Portion Size vs. Serving Size

Before we dive into the positives that come with portion control, let's first nail down the difference between portion size and serving size. These terms are often used interchangeably, but they're not the same thing, according to the National Institutes of Health (NIH).

The difference is simple: A portion size is an amount you eat, big or small, and a serving size is the amount of food you should be eating. A serving size is a standard set by a food's nutrition label, while portion size varies depending on who's dishing out the fare.

Serving sizes are most often measured out in cups or ounces. For example, one 6-ounce steak is usually considered a standard portion, but two servings of meat, according to the U.S. Department of Agriculture.

An easy way to learn portion control is to compare food portion sizes to everyday objects. For example, a serving of baked potato is the size of your fist, and a serving of peanut butter is the size of a ping-pong ball, per the NIH.

According to the Centers for Disease Control and Prevention, the more food you're served, the more you will likely eat. So, while you adjust to eating smaller portions, switch to smaller plates, which will make your portions appear larger (and hey, you eat with your eyes first, right?). This is a small change that can make the process a little bit less daunting.

Health Benefits of Eating Smaller Portions

Better Blood Sugar Control

Your body turns the foods you eat — especially carbohydrates — into glucose, a type of sugar that serves as your body's primary Source of energy. When you eat a large portion of food, your glucose levels rise quickly. When your bloodstream is flooded with glucose, your pancreas releases insulin to move that glucose into your cells for use.

But the faster glucose levels rise, the more likely it is that your pancreas will produce too much insulin in response, leading to low blood sugar. As a result, your brain is tricked into thinking you need more glucose, and you start to feel hungry, often with a sugar craving. You can avoid this negative cycle of high and low blood sugar — which can lead to weight gain — by eating small, frequent meals, which will help keep your glucose and insulin levels stable.

Increased Satiety and Weight Control

Eating smaller portions can curb cravings and help reduce overall calorie intake. Feeling satiated, or having a feeling of fullness, can affect how much you eat and how often you eat.

The British Nutrition Foundation suggests eating slowly and with smaller portions to feel more satiated after a meal.

Eating smaller portions also allows your body to use the food you eat immediately for energy, instead of storing the excess as fat. Losing weight isn't as simple as only controlling your portion sizes, but when you learn to watch the amount of food you eat, you can begin to practice mindful eating, which can help you make healthier food choices, according to Harvard Health Publishing.

Things That Happen When You Eat Too Fast — and How to Slow Down

Improved Digestion

Many of us have been there: That moment when you're done with Thanksgiving dinner and suddenly regret eating as much as you did. Once a year might not be a big deal, but regularly eating large portions can wreak havoc on your digestive system.

Having larger portion sizes makes your stomach stretch further and causes it to push against your other organs, which can lead to a lot of discomforts. You also run the risk of having heartburn because having a full stomach can push hydrochloric acid back up into your esophagus. Finally, you also may produce excess gas from that big meal, which is never a good feeling.

Money Back in Your Pocket

Eating smaller portions can also result in financial benefits, especially when it comes to dining out.

For example, one way to practice portion control at restaurants is to order kid-sized meals, which are generally less expensive than adult meals and closer to the correct serving size you should be eating.

Adult portion sizes at restaurants can equal two, three or more servings. So, here's a pro tip: When the food is delivered to your table, ask your server for a take-away container and immediately remove at least half the food from your plate. By taking 50 percent of your entree home, you'll be getting two meals for the price of one.

It is all about discipline. By counting every calorie and logging your exercise hours, you can stay firmly on track while understanding how each contributes to your weight loss goals.

For example, if you adhere to your diet, you can see if certain activities, such as swimming or biking, help you lose weight faster than others. This allows you to find out what works best for you as an individual.

Let's Start This Diet

First of all, this is not a crash diet or a regular diet.

This is the long-term, steady lifestyle diet designed for those of us with over fifty pounds to lose. If you are looking for a crash diet or a regular diet, please refer to the first 32 pages. Let's begin. You don't need to take notes; you can always refer back to this guide.

I have researched a dozen of the most effective diets I could find on the market and have cheery picked the methods that worked best. I have also made this diet the most comfortable, most simple diet to accomplish.

Most Diets Fail, Not This One

No one plans to fail their diet, and no one suddenly decides to quit their diet. Diets become boring without motivation, and we don't feel the need to keep suffering because we don't see much of an improvement. My "Life Diet" works differently than any other diet plan. You eat the foods you usually eat; only your portion size is smaller. Here is the logic behind this system.

- Assuming your weight is legally steady right now (it doesn't change more than ten pounds, up or down), the actual portion size of every meal you eat is what we are locked-on to. Forget calories, and continually weighing yourself, keeping track of what, when, etc., those things are why other diets fail, we aren't interested in any of those things, we are going to alter our eating lifestyle, to a point, we don't even think about it anymore, folks will start telling you, you're looking so much better. You will know why, and it will cause you to keep going, perhaps even starting to replace some of the unhealthy foods you eat now.

- If you decrease the actual size of each meal you eat and make no other changes at all, your weight will slowly begin to drop, and if you adjust your meal portion size, and if you do any of the things I recommend in the first 32 pages of this book, you will increase the speed of your weight loss.

- One thing NOT included with those other diets (and it is the reason most diets fail) is motivation; I SOLVED that, with regular, weekly videos for you to watch, and feel some motivation. Many other people, just like you, are starting this diet with me, simultaneously, on December 1st, and you can start it at any time afterward, on your own, and use the same videos to help you with your motivation at your own pace.

THE LIFESTYLE CHANGE

There are three types of eating problems, "Eaters," three meals, and a few snacks. "Grazers," they eat when they are hungry, but not many snacks. The third type is the most dangerous, unhealthiest, most challenging weight to control, called "Greeters," they eat at least three meals a day, with snacks, whenever they want, all day long.

Most of us who have failed at many diets are "Greeters." We're friendly folks, but we find it impossible to get a handle on these love handles, UNTIL NOW.

Both "Eaters" and "Grazers" can lose weight by applying the systems, calorie counting; in the first 32 pages, "Greaters," however, need to adjust their eating lifestyle functionally. This section is for "Greeters," and if you follow these recommendations, you will not only lose weight, but you will continue to lose weight, slowly, but continuously, so, at any given time, a week later, you will weigh less than the week, before.

Imagine the joy you will feel from trying on an old favorite shirt and finding it fits great, or trying on some old pants you gave up on ever wearing again, and there's room inside. This will be if you follow the set rules.

The Life Diet

I reviewed a dozen diet plans and cherry-picked those methods which were most useful from each.

The most difficult diets are the first diets to fail, so we simplify everything

Step One

Start measuring the size of the portions of food you are currently eating for a few weeks before starting the diet.

Look at the portion size of the meals you eat now; the secret to this diet is to reduce your typical portion size. This is the actual size of your portions on your plate.

There are several ways to measure your current, average portion size.

You can use a small scale to weigh your portions.

You can use a spoon to measure your portions by counting the spoonfuls (always use the same size spoon).

You could use a measuring cup.

You can use plates with dividers built into them.

You can use your mind to estimate how many scoops of food is there if the scoop is your four fingers (without using your thumb). This is the way to go; z

Once you are confident, you can estimate the standard portion sizes of your food you are currently eating, now, Begin the diet.

The "Life Diet."

At EVERY meal, from now on, you will:

Drink a small cup of water directly before you dish out your meal. Get used to doing it. Doing so will help you slowly shrink your stomach's size, and if you start to enjoy the results, you can increase the size of the cup later on.

Decrease your average portion size of each meal you are eating by 25-35 percent.

You can calculate all this out, but why bother? You can estimate by merely using your mind to picture what size a four-finger, the scoop is, then changing it to three fingers.

If it's more comfortable and use something else to measure with, cut the amount by 25-35 percent of each (non-fruit or vegetable) product you put on the plate. You can eat all the fruit and vegetables you want.

The diet works as a straightforward, mathematical equation, given the constant quantities of your current caloric intake, minus, (25-35 percent).

That's how the diet works.

If you follow this plan for every meal, you will begin losing 1-2 pounds per week.

You will want to start tweaking the diet a little. Your goal should be set at two pounds per week.

Trying to lose over 2 pounds per week will cause you to fail. Losing weight takes time, just like it did, gaining it.

If you are losing over two pounds per week, you can modify your caloric intake in several ways. The easiest method is to cut back the amount of water in your cup. Congruently, you can increase the amount of water in the cup to increase your weekly weight loss.

Communicate with others

To succeed with this diet, you will need to seek others' help who are dieting. I suggest my vlog series on YouTube called "Bob's World Life," where I will be talking about the diet, as I begin it, on January 1st. 2021. I hope you will begin the diet with me and keep watching the diet updates. I will be posting.

If you want to join in with the fun, you can. You don't need to tell anyone your starting weight or your current weight; it is not essential to anyone but you. In our discussions, we are only concerned with the amount of weight you have lost to date.

The rest is up to you; when you are ready, go to YouTube, and subscribe to Bob's World life", and watch, as I post a new video each week. I will number the vlogs by week number, in case you start the diet after I do, so you can watch the week number that matches your diet schedule as we do this together.

I look forward to joining me with this diet; this might save both of our lives.

www.ingramcontent.com/pod-product-compliance
Lightning Source LLC
Chambersburg PA
CBHW070825220526
45466CB00002B/757